The Revolutionary Leptin Resistance Guide

All You Need To Know About Preventing Or Reversing Leptin Resistance To Lose Weight Immediately

Table of Contents

Introduction

This book contains proven steps and strategies on how to eat healthy and lose weight based on the prevention and reversion of leptin resistance.

If you are interested in discovering everything there is to know about leptin resistance, this guide is the essential resource for you to read. It will teach you the healthy eating choices for losing weight, based on the prevention and reversion of leptin resistance.

Here Is A Preview Of What You'll Learn...

- How important is the leptin hormone for the human body

- What is leptin resistance and how it can affect you

- How to organize your diet and prevent/reverse the leptin resistance

- The role of physical exercise in reducing the leptin resistance

- The best weight loss plan for those who have developed leptin resistance

- Healthy recipes to lose all that extra weight

- Top things to remember about leptin resistance

- The rules of the leptin diet

- Much, much more!

Chapter 1 – The importance of leptin for the human body and leptin-resistance

Not many people know that for a fact, but leptin is actually one of the most important hormones of the human body. If you pay attention to the important role this hormone plays, you could change your health and lose all that extra, stubborn weight. Apart from the weight management, leptin can influence the functioning of the endocrine glands (especially the thyroid), the reproductive process and even the cardiovascular health. Studies have shown a connection between leptin and the functioning of the brain (mental capacity). Leptin also regulates the stress levels, influencing inflammatory processes and having an effect over the immune system as well.

Unfortunately, the leptin hormone has only recently been given the proper attention. Produced in the adipose tissue, meaning in the stored fat, it seems to be more than a hormone but rather a metabolic organ, with a clear influence over the thyroid and adrenal glands. When leptin is released from the stored fat, it travels through the bloodstream to the brain, providing information on how much energy the rest of the body has. Upon receiving the signal from the leptin hormone, the brain will activate the metabolism and promote the consumption of fat for energy. When you have eaten enough quantities of food, the leptin hormone will rise, sending the full signal to the brain (you can look at the whole process as the leptin gauge providing information about the available fuel in the body).

Being overweight also means that you might be experiencing a broken leptin gauge, thus feeling the constant need to eat more food in order to feel satisfied (no full signal reaches the brain). If the leptin gauge would function normally, the brain would receive the satiety signal and would activate the metabolism, promoting the consumption of excess weight. On the other hand, in case the leptin levels are too low, a signal will be transmitted to the brain and the metabolic rate is going to be reduced (in many ways, this process can be compared to hibernation).

There is one more thing that you should know about leptin and the leptin gauge. Compulsive eating is often encountered in those who are overweight, as these people have grown accustomed to ignoring the full signal. When one constantly ignores this signal, it is only normal that the leptin gauge will eventually become broken and the obesity is going to become worse.

Leptin is one of the essential hormones that work to regulate the brain function, especially in relation to the satiety sensation and the activation/deactivation of the metabolism. What you need to remember is that leptin also has an effect on the immune system and on the activity of the other glands, including the thyroid, the adrenal glands and the reproductive glands. If the leptin gauge is broken, apart from the excess weight, one will also suffer from other hormonal dysfunctions, not being able to manage stress in an effective manner.

In overweight people, the production of leptin occurs in excessive quantities, as the hormone constantly tries to warn the brain about the 'full' sensation. When too much leptin is produced at the level of the body, this also means that the person will enter into a vicious cycle. The extra weight is going to lead to increased quantities of leptin, these having a negative effect on the actual functioning of the leptin hormone. This vicious cycle leads to the development of leptin resistance, with a negative impact on the brain and its capacity to activate or de-activate the metabolism, in accordance to the information sent by the leptins stored in the adipose tissue.

Leptin resistance might not be something you know by the name but, once you analyze the clear facts, it might easier to decide whether you are having this problem or not. If you constantly obsess about food, thinking about what you are going to eat next and always finding excuses to eat foods that are clearly bad for you, this might mean that you have developed leptin resistance. You have basically come to the point where you live to eat and not the other way around.

In order to understand the way leptin resistance develops, you can think about the patients who have been diagnosed with type 2 diabetes. These are the patients who have developed insulin resistance – this means that their pancreas produces insulin in high quantities but the body simply fails to respond properly to these changes, leading to a wide range of upsetting symptoms. The same thing happens in those who have developed leptin resistance – the brain does not respond to the full signal anymore, leading to obesity. The higher the levels of leptin are, the more weight will be added to the body. This is practically a paradox – as the brain is starved, the body becomes more obese.

In healthy individuals, when the leptin levels are too low, the brain will perceive the food as even more rewarding than it normally is. On the other hand, when the leptin levels are high, the reward system is not that powerful and one experiences the satiety sensation. In the situation that a person has developed leptin resistance, the reward system does not function properly and it does not provide the person with the satiety sensation. Even though the leptin levels increase and increase, the person does not feel like he/she is full, continuing to eat. The fact that no information is offered to the brain in regard to the fullness is one of the major factors contributing to obesity. When the brain does not get the leptin signal, that is when excess weight starts to gather and obesity becomes a problem.

As you will see in the following chapters, it is possible to prevent and even to reverse the leptin resistance. So, do not worry, as the sun will come out on your street as well. You just need to learn how to be in harmony with the leptin hormone and fix that broken gauge, discovering once again the right way to eat.

Chapter 2 – The leptin diet and its most important rules

If you are overweight, you have probably tried every diet, without being able to obtain the desired results. However, it's never too late to change and choose a lifestyle that is both healthy and efficient when it comes to the weight loss. The leptin resistance can be prevented and reversed by choosing the leptin diet, which is more of a lifestyle change than an actual diet. It will help you keep the leptin hormone in control, losing all that extra weight and enjoying the renewed levels of energy, as well as the improved health. With the leptin diet, there are three things that are highly important: the quality of the food, the moment when you eat and the quantity you eat. The secret of this lifestyle change is that you watch out for what you eat and draw your energy from good sources.

Unlike other diets, the leptin diet provides guaranteed results, helping you not only to lose that extra weight but also to maintain the current diet for the rest of your life. You will finally be able to enjoy life to the fullest, feeling filled with energy and vitality. The leptin diet has a positive effect over the metabolism, keeping the blood sugar under control and guaranteeing an optimal health status. However, if you want for this lifestyle change to provide you with the above-mentioned results, there are certain rules that you will have to abide. Let's check them out!

The first and most important rule is that you never eat after dinner, making sure that you eat the last meal of the day with at least three hours before going to bed. The proposers of this diet consider that there should be at least 11-12 hours between your supper and the breakfast of next day. This means that you should never go to bed with a full stomach, making sure that you eat an early dinner.

Why is so important that you follow this rule? Well, let's find out a bit more information on the leptin and its mechanism of action. First of all, you should know that the leptin functions in accordance to the circadian rhythm, with the leptin levels being at their highest point in the evening. This also means that the leptin hormones are most active during the night, when they contribute to the regulatory and reparatory processed in different parts of the body. They play an essential role in the metabolism of melatonin but also in the functioning of other hormones, making sure that the sleep has its rejuvenating properties.

During sleep, the leptin hormones are actively involved in the burning of the fat deposits, a process which occurs naturally. If you go to bed on a full stomach, you will prevent the activity of the leptins and hence the weight gain will occur. Following your cravings is not a good idea, especially when it comes to those that appear in the evening or even during the night. When a person experiences cravings, this is a clear sign that the leptin gauge has malfunctioned. You need to be stronger than your cravings and exert your self-control, making sure that you do not eat after the early dinner.

The second rule of the leptin diet is that you eat three meals each and every day. In order to lose weight and revert the leptin resistance, you must allow for at least five or six hours to pass between the meals, without any snacks in between. The period between the meals is essential, as this is the moment when fat is eliminated from the blood circulation. If you eat constantly, the triglycerides are going to build up in the blood, having a negative impact on the activity of the leptin at the level of the brain. Due to the leptin resistance, the brain cannot provide feedback to the rest of the body, meaning there will be no satiety sensation.

The human body is a perfectly designed machine, with specific times for eating. Even though the human body has evolved, we are still not equipped for constant eating. When one eats all the time, the metabolism is confused and the leptin hormone no longer provides the brain with the necessary information. You start eating more than you need and end up accumulating extra weight.

There are a lot of misconceptions about eating and one of the most important ones is actually related to snacking. It is a false notion that you need a snack between meals, in order to keep your blood sugar at stable levels. On the contrary, if you keep on snacking, you will lead to the malfunctioning of the leptin hormone and thus to the weight gain. Between meals, the liver is active, contributing to the elimination of the triglycerides from the blood. You need this pause between the meals, so as to get rid of the extra fat. If you avoid snacks, you will also benefit from an improvement in the mechanism of the leptin. Thus, the fat that has been stored in different parts of the body (such as the hips or the thighs) is going to be burned during sleeping and the weight loss process is going to be successful.

The third rule of the leptin diet is that you pay increased attention to the portion size of each meal. When you are hungry, you might have the tendency to eat until you are full but you also need to remember that the brain does not receive this information only until it is too late. If you want to reverse the leptin resistance, you need to start reducing the portion size and also to finish a meal when you are less than full. There is a saying that goes something like that: "always leave the table when you are still a little bit hungry".

When we eat, the brain receives the full signal from the leptins approximately after twenty minutes. This is why it is also important to eat slowly and chew your food thoroughly, so as to avoid overeating to feel full. Listen to what your body is trying to tell you and stop when you receive the full signal. One of the biggest mistakes is ignoring that signal and continuing to eat, a mistake that is often the cause of obesity.

Taking a look at other populations, such as the French or the Chinese, you can easily understand why they do not have a problem with obesity. Not only are their food choices a lot healthier but they also tend to eat portions that are smaller in size. Unfortunately, the fast food industry promotes the bigger portions at cheaper prices, so you are always encouraged to eat more. You have to fight this temptation and become accustomed to smaller portions, with healthy food choices. Unless you have a very demand job (from a physical point of view), there is no excuse to fill your plate to the max.

You need to provide your body with food that is healthy, including all the major food groups and not just filling your plate with high quantities of food. This leads us to another important rule of the leptin diet, which states that one should never skip breakfast and that this meal should include a high protein intake. You might not be aware of this fact but, by choosing proteins for your breakfast, you will boost your metabolism. The activation of the metabolism is possible by choosing good sources of proteins and it can be as high as 30%, burning all that extra fat. Instead, if you choose a breakfast that is high in carbs, you will feel tired and these are going to be easily deposited as fat in different parts of the body.

It is said that the best moment to make a change is now. You need to forget about your usual breakfast habits, such as cereals, waffles and bagels – all of these are sources of carbs and they are not healthy breakfast choices. This is valid for all those who are struggling to lose all that extra weight and in particular for middle-aged individuals. The carbs eaten in the morning are going to have a negative impact over your energy levels, leaving you craving for a snack soon after the meal.

How do you know if your breakfast choices are not good? Well, just think about the period until it is time for lunch. If you are having a hard time concentrating and you feel like you do not have enough energy, this means that your breakfast choices are not that good. Cravings and energy crashes are signs that you are not feeding your body with the right food, with a negative influence on the leptin mechanism. Among the healthy choices that you can consider for breakfast, be sure to include eggs, cottage cheese and other similar products. The important thing is that you choose good sources of protein and include them in your daily breakfast.

The last rule of the leptin diet is that you reduce your carbohydrate intake, not only for breakfast, but also for the other meals of the day. However, this does not mean that you should cut out the carbs completely. Keep in mind that carbs provide you with immediate energy and that you need them, but only in moderate quantities. Without carbs, you will suffer from thyroid dysfunction, the electrolytes are going to become imbalanced and your muscle will become weaker. At the same time, there will be a negative impact on the other hormones and also on the fat burning process.

In case you are struggling with extra weight, you need to pay increased attention to the quantities of carbs you are eating. In order to lose weight, you will have to stay organized and arrange your meals, so as to have an equal part of proteins and carbs with each portion. There is no need to calculate the number of calories and you can add fresh, vegetables that are rich in fiber to all meals. Among the best sources of protein, there are: chicken, turkey and eggs. As for carbs, consider the following foods: bread, rice, pasta, potatoes and corn. You can also take soluble fiber supplements, in order to obtain the satiety sensation but avoid filling up on carbs.

In conclusion, the leptin diet is the perfect choice for those who want to lose weight. As long as you follow the above-mentioned rules, you will be able to lose all that extra weight and reverse the negative consequences of the leptin resistance. Keep in mind that the leptin diet can also be a great lifestyle choice, even if you are not suffering from excess weight. The healthy choices, along with the rules, will guarantee the prevention of leptin resistance and ensure a status of optimal health for the rest of your life.

Chapter 3 – How to organize your diet to prevent or reverse leptin resistance

From what has been said so far, you have probably understood that you can prevent or reverse the consequences of leptin resistance by changing your eating habits, including the moments when you eat and the actual foods that are part of your diet. The new diet should include fresh foods, preferably those that have been organically grown – these will provide your body with the necessary

energy and also promote the weight loss process. At the same time, it is essential to eliminate any foods that have chemicals, artificial substances or sweeteners, as these are quite harmful. You need to start eating real foods, making sure that each meal is satisfying and delicious, sending the correct signals to your brain (in regard to the satiety sensation).

In terms of calories, it is important that you try to maintain within a reasonable amount for each meal, without obsessing about a specific number. In general, it is recommended that you keep each meal between 400 and 600 calories, with the following proportions being respected for each meal: 40% fat, 30% carbs and 30% proteins. If you are looking for precise quantities to eat for each day, you should consume proteins in a quantity between 50 and 75% of your ideal body weight (per day). As for the fiber intake, this should vary between 30 and 50 grams per day (if your diet does not provide sufficient quantities of fiber, you can increase your daily intake with the help of fiber supplements).

No matter how accustomed you might have been to snacking between meals, it is essential that you give this habit up. It is very important that you avoid the snacks that you are used to eating a couple of hours after your breakfast or lunch, as these will interfere with the leptin activity and provide the brain with the wrong signals. If you want to lose weight, you will have to concentrate on the three basic meals, meaning breakfast, lunch and dinner. As it was already mentioned, between the meals, the liver will be active, cleaning the blood of the triglycerides and contributing to the fat burning process.

When it comes to beverages, you have to concentrate on those that have no calories and a natural taste. It is clear that you are not allowed to consume beverages that contain artificial sweeteners, as these can have a harmful effect on the blood sugar levels and also on the leptin activity. The recommended choices for beverages include water (you can add lemon slices for a fresh taste), tea (depending on the season, you can drink it warm or with ice) and coffee (black, no sugar).

Apart from the drinks that contain artificial sweeteners, you should also exclude the following from your diet: sodas (including diet sodas, as these contain artificial sweeteners as well), flavored waters and energy drinks of all kinds. It is also recommended that you avoid both the drinks and the foods that are made from soy, as these can have an irritating effect on the thyroid gland and even inhibit the fat burning process (negative impact on the weight loss process).

At first, it will not be easy to make all these changes and eliminate foods that you have grown accustomed to throughout the years. You might be quite hungry between the meals, feeling the urgency to eat your common snacks. Without the snacking, at the beginning, you will experience energy slumps and want to go back to old habits. This is the moment when you want to resist and enforce your self-control – think about your health and how badly you want to lose weight.

If you are feeling hungry, do not be quick to rush to food (especially if there is still a lot of time until the next meal). Instead, drink a glass of water. When a person has developed leptin resistance, the brain might have a hard time making the difference between the hunger and the thirst signal. By drinking a glass of water, you will be able to delay the hunger sensation and also hydrate your body. If you still cannot ward off hunger in between the meals, it is recommended that you take leptin supplements instead of snacks. These will regulate the hunger sensation, helping you resist until the next meal. You can also consider taking these supplements between lunch and dinner, in order to counteract the effects of the afternoon energy slump (caused by the lack of snacking as well).

In general, between the meals, it is recommended that you keep yourself busy. If you are work, things are going to be easier, as you can concentrate on the things that you have to do. However, when you are at home, you might find it harder to stay from temptations, especially if you need to prepare the meals for the rest of your family. Try to include as many activities as you can in your day, preferably away from food. During this period, it is important to be physically active, so you may want to pick up a sport or go to a gym. The physical movement is benefic for the weight loss process and it will also cause the release of endorphins, which are considered as the happiness hormones.

In regard to the nutritional supplements, these can be quite helpful for adapting to the new lifestyle change. As long as you choose nutritional supplements that include only natural and top-quality ingredients, you do not have to worry about anything else. The leptin supplements are highly recommended, as they have a lot of positive effects on your body, such as: activation of the metabolism, correction of hormonal imbalance, elimination of food cravings and hunger sensation. As you will start taking the nutritional supplements instead of your snacks, you will notice that you have increased energy. The energy given by these supplements is going to allow you to stay on track and reach your ideal weight. Just keep in mind that these supplements should be taken with plenty of water. Their main benefit is that they reduce your vulnerability towards bad foods or less healthy food choices; they also impact the tendency to overeat, which is another definite advantage to be considered.

Chapter 4 – The role of physical exercise in reducing leptin resistance

The fact that leptin is a hormone which is synthesized by the adipose tissue is no longer news. The satiety hormone plays a number of roles in the human body, regulating the levels of energy and also the metabolism. Leptin has the power to influence weight, in a good or a bad sense, as you have already discovered. If you have decided to reverse the leptin resistance, you should know that physical exercise can be of tremendous importance.

Studies have shown that physical exercise can have a significant contribution in decreasing the concentration of leptin. The benefits of physical exercise have been known for a long time but it was only recently that a connection has been found between obesity, leptin resistance and active movement. The beneficial effect over the leptin resistance doubles with the one of decreasing insulin levels, helping people lose excessive weight in an efficient manner. Combined with a healthy diet, physical exercise can be the best weapon against leptin resistance and obesity.

The interesting thing about physical exercise is that it leads to lower leptin concentrations immediately after each session. The leptin concentrations continue to be lowered during the next couple of days, which is suggestive of the fact that regular physical exercise might be beneficial on a long term basis as well. A study has demonstrate the beneficial effects of physical exercise in overweight, post-menopausal women. The study has showed a reduced concentration of leptin in the women taking part in the research, after half an hour of physical exercise.

It seems that physical exercise is able to influence the circadian rhythm of leptin, thus reducing the leptin resistance and allowing for the fat burning processes to occur in a natural manner. Being physically activate, you also regulate the activity of the hormones that have an influence on the leptin concentration, such as the cortisol or the growth hormone. By regulating all the hormones at the level of different glands, you can lose all those extra pounds and reach the ideal weight you have always dreamt of.

Resistance exercises are highly recommended as a form of physical exercise, as they have been shown to provide a significant reduction of the leptin concentration in the blood. Among the exercises that you can perform, there are: squats, bench presses, leg presses and lateral pull downs. Keep in mind that the benefits of the resistance exercises are mostly related to the activation of the metabolism, the weight loss being promoted almost instantly.

When considering physical exercise for weight loss purposes, you also have to think about your current level of fitness. Overweight people generally avoid physical movement, due to the tremendous effort the simplest movements require. However, it is important that you start with small steps and progress to higher amounts of effort with each day that passes. This might not be an easy thing to accomplish but you have to find your inner motivation and work out, so as to reverse the effects of the leptin resistance.

In healthy individuals, who have a weight that is within the normal standard, the most significant reduction of leptin concentration has been identified after they have taken part in sports such as marathon running or skiing. This just goes to prove that endurance exercises, depending on your potential level of effort, might help you in losing weight.

The leptin concentration can also be reduced in significant quantities by performing physical exercise for a longer period of time (over an hour of training). In the beginning, you might not be able to sustain such a long period of exercise but, with the passing of time, you might be able to increase the duration of the training session. The reason why you need to think about long-term exercise is that it has the possibility to reduce the circulating leptin, promoting at the same time the regulation of hormonal imbalances in different glands of the body.

Long-duration exercises are extremely beneficial for those who are experiencing the negative effects of leptin resistance. In choosing the exercises that can have an impact over the leptin activity, you will also have to take into consideration the following: current level of fitness, other pre-existing conditions (especially heart disease) and the diet you have chosen to lose weight.

There are many benefits of physical exercise for those who are overweight, whether we are talking about the reduction of the adipose tissue, the balancing of the hormone concentrations and the cleaning of the blood from fatty metabolites, such as triglycerides. But the biggest benefit remains related to the modification of the leptin response. By lowering the leptin concentrations, physical exercise might be one of the most valuable weapons you have, helping you lose weight and have a fantastic figure.

Chapter 5 – Say goodbye to leptin resistance with the weight loss plan

Starting a new diet can be a challenging experience, as it requires that you give up bad habits and concentrate on making healthy eating choices. As you have discovered by now, obesity is caused by leptin resistance and it can be very difficult, if not impossible, to lose weight without choosing the foods that eliminate this problem. The good news is that this weight loss plan has the reduction of leptin resistance as its main objective, helping you keep your appetite under control and eliminating all that extra weight. By following the recommendations made for this weight loss plan, you will be able to activate your metabolism and maintain the ideal weight for the rest of your life.

Before diving into the phases of the weight loss plan, it is important to mention that not all diets are healthy. You should definitely avoid the crash diets, as these can have negative effects on your health. The reason why these diets are so detrimental to your health is actually related to the impact they have on the leptin mechanism – without providing your body with the necessary nutrients, the leptin hormone goes into what is known as the "starvation mode".

As soon as you start going back to your bad eating habits, you will gain all the weight you have lost with the crash diet.

What makes this weight loss plan different? Just follow the phases that are recommended below and you will soon see the weight loss results, without worrying about any side-effects. Apart from that, this weight loss plan has the ability to reduce and revert the negative consequences of leptin resistance, helping you maintain the ideal weight for the rest of your life. So, if you are ready to lose that extra weight, there is no better moment than the present to go ahead with this weight loss plan.

The first phase of the weight loss lasts for approximately four days but it can be extended or even doubled if necessary. During these first days, your meals are going to consist of protein powders and fiber supplements. These can be consumed as beverages, being mixed with one of the following: water, fruit or vegetable juice or different types of milk (regular, rice or almond milk are allowed; avoid soy milk, as it can have a negative influence over the functioning of the thyroid). These beverages are going to cover your meals for the next three days, acting as a substitute for breakfast, lunch and dinner.

During these three days, you are also allowed to add a fruit serving to the protein/fiber mix. If you want, you can consume the fruit serving fresh, immediately after the protein/fiber mix. After breakfast or lunch, you can also drink a cup of coffee or tea (however, such beverages are not allowed at dinner). While you are allowed to add cream to your coffee or tea, you must refrain from adding sugar or artificial sweeteners to these beverages. Also, it is absolutely forbidden to have any snacks between the meals (no night indulgences as well).

At first, it may be difficult to follow this weight loss plan, especially during the afternoon or at night, when the cravings kick in. This is the best time to show yours self-control and regain control over your own body. If you last these few days, without breaking the rules, soon you will notice that you no longer experience such intense cravings. On the fourth day of the weight loss plan, you are allowed to have a regular dinner – however, you will have to make sure that the number of calories ranges between 400 and 500 calories. The dinner should include lean meat or cottage cheese (as a source of proteins), combined with veggies and carbs. In regard to dessert, you can have only a small bite or, preferably, none (depending on your willpower once more).

The main purpose of this dinner is to help you experience the full signal. If the leptin-resistance is not severe, the above-mentioned dinner should provide you with a satiety signal from the leptin hormone. If you will not experience the satiety sensation, it is recommended that you repeat the first four days of the weight loss plan, with its protein/fiber mix meals and fruits. Once again, on the fourth day, you have to repeat the satiety test. The moment you receive the correct signal from the leptin hormone, you can proceed to the second phase of the weight loss plan.

The second phase lasts for approximately two weeks, requiring that you make two very important decisions – first, how much weight you want to lose and, second, how fast do you want for such a thing to happen. During the second phase, you will maintain the protein/fiber mix meal for breakfast and lunch. For dinner, you are allowed to have a regular dinner, consisting of 400-500 calories as well. There is an alternative mode in which the second phase can develop – you can stick with the three protein/fiber mix meals per day, eating the regular dinner every other day or on the third day. What happens if you eat more than the number of recommended calories? Well, the answer is simple. You need to consume all those extra calories by getting more physically active in your next training session. The important thing is that you do not give up and return to bad eating habits.

For the third phase of the weight loss plan, you can stick with just one protein/fiber mix meal per day and eat two regular meals. The important thing is that you do not go over the recommended 400-500 calories for each meal. You will see that these meals provide you with all the energy you need, with a guaranteed full signal as well. You will no longer feel the urgency to overeat, especially in the afternoon or during the night. Thanks to the reduced need for snacking or overeating, you will lose all those extra pounds and finally reach your ideal weight. However, if it happens that you have gone off track and returned to the bad eating patterns, you must go back to the second or even the first phase.

Chapter 6 – Healthy recipes that reduce leptin resistance

As you have seen in the last chapter, the leptin diet requires that you replace your meals with protein and fiber mixes for the first few days. After that, you are allowed to eat regular food for dinner. As you progress with the diet, you will be able to eat more meals of regular food, containing healthy choices and helping you maintain your ideal weight. In this chapter, you can find several delicious recipes – these recipes only contain healthy choices, so as to prevent or revert the effects of leptin resistance over your body.

These are some of the most delicious recipes you can consider for losing weight:

- *Coconut rice with grilled shrimp*
    - Ingredients required – olive oil (2 tbsp.), white onion (1, diced), red/yellow peppers (2, diced), garlic cloves (6), ginger (1 tsp., fresh, minced), tomatoes (2, peeled, diced), coconut (1/4 cup, grated), basmati rice (1 ¾ cups), water (3 cups), yogurt (1 cup, low fat), parsley

(1/2 cup, chopped), shrimp (16-20), salt and pepper to taste

- o Preparation – start by sautéing the onion and the peppers. Add the garlic and the ginger to the mix, followed by the tomatoes and the coconut. Cook for approximately five minutes and then add the basmati rice, stirring frequently for about two minutes. After that, you add the water and let it boil. Reduce the heat and let the whole mixture simmer for about 20 minutes. Remove the mixture from the heat and add the yoghurt to the mixture. Grill the shrimp using wooden skewers and enjoy.

- Chicken cutlets with cherry salsa
  - o Ingredients required – cherries (2 cups), white onion (1/2 cup, chopped), tomato (1, chopped), salt (3/4 tsp.), black pepper (1/2 tsp.), cilantro (2 tbsp., fresh, chopped), breadcrumbs (3/4 cup, whole wheat), chicken

cutlets (4, boneless and skinless), olive oil (2 tbsp., extra-virgin)

- ○ Preparation – start by adding the cherries together with the chopped onion, tomato, salt and pepper into a blender. Add the cilantro and let it aside. Take the breadcrumbs and make sure that you coat the chicken with them (adding a little bit of salt and pepper as well). Cook the chicken cutlets on each side, until they turn golden. Enjoy with cherry salsa on the top.

- Lentil and quinoa salad
    - ○ Ingredients required – lentils (1 cup), salt (2 tsp.), quinoa (1 cup), balsamic vinegar (3 tbsp.), extra virgin olive oil (3 tbsp.), sea salt (2 tsp.), plum tomato (1, diced), avocado (1, diced), cilantro (2 tsp., diced), lemon zest (2 tbsp.)
    - ○ Preparation – start by boiling the lentils in salted water. In a separate pot, cook the quinoa, using salt as well. Drain the lentils

and the quinoa and add them into a bowl, letting them to cool. Prepare the dressing for the salad by mixing the olive oil with the balsamic vinegar. Add the chopped tomato and avocado to the lentil & quinoa mixture. You can use the cilantro and lemon zest, as well as the vinaigrette, in order to freshen up the taste of the salad.

- Fruit smoothie
  - Ingredients required – almond milk (1 cup), pineapple (1 cup), coconut (1 tsp.), blueberries (1/2 cup), protein powder (1 scoop)
  - Preparation – add all the above mentioned ingredients into your blender and process them until they are thoroughly mixed. Pour the contents into a large glass and enjoy.

- Kale smoothie
  - Ingredients required – pear (1/2), avocado (1/4), lemon (1/2), cilantro (1 tsp.), kale (1

cup), ginger (1/2 tsp., grated), coconut water (1/2 cup), protein powder (1 scoop).

- o Preparation - add all the above mentioned ingredients into your blender and process them until they are thoroughly mixed. Pour the contents into a large glass and enjoy.

- Mango & avocado salad
    - o Ingredients required – jalapeno chili (1/2, minced), lime juice (1/2 cup), olive oil (1/4 cup), sea salt (1/2 tsp.), pepper (to taste), mango (1), avocado (1), organic salad greens (6 cups)
    - o Preparation – start by preparing the dressing for the salad. For the dressing, mix the jalapeno chili with the lime juice. Add the olive oil, salt and pepper. Cut the avocado and mango in large chunks. Add the salad greens into a large bowl, with the avocado and mango. For the last step, add the salad dressing and enjoy.

- Turkey burger

  - Ingredients required – ground turkey (1 pound), marinara sauce (1 cup), Gouda cheese (1/4 cup), mozzarella cheese (1/4 cup), pita/burger bun, organic salad greens (topping), red onion (1/2 cup, chopped), salt and pepper to taste

  - Preparation – mix the ground turkey with the marinara sauce, the Gouda and mozzarella cheese, adding salt and pepper to taste. Split the meat into four servings and cook it on the grill. Place the turkey burger in the bun or on the pita, topping it with red onion and organic salad greens. Enjoy!

- Greek salad

  - Ingredients required – red wine vinegar (1/3 cup), extra virgin olive oil (2 tbsp.), oregano (1 tbsp.), garlic powder (1 tsp.), salt (1/4 tsp.), pepper (1/4 tsp.), baby spinach (6 cups), chicken (12 oz.), tomatoes (2, diced), cucumber (1, chopped), red onion (1/2 cup), black olives (1/2 cup), feta cheese (1/2 cup)

- Preparation – start by cooking the chicken and letting it aside to cool down. Prepare the dressing for the salad by mixing the following ingredients together: vinegar, oil, oregano, garlic powder, salt and pepper. Take a large bowl and add the cooked chicken, together with baby spinach, tomatoes, cucumber, onion, olives and feta cheese. Add the salad dressing and enjoy.

- Salmon fillet with asparagus
  - Ingredients required – salmon fillet (4), rosemary (1 tbsp.), salt (1 tsp.), asparagus (1 ½ pounds), extra virgin olive oil (1 ½ tbsp.), onion (1, diced), pine nuts (2 tbsp.), water (1 cup), brown rice (1/2 cup)
  - Preparation – start by seasoning the salmon with salt and rosemary. Leave it aside for one hour. Cook the brown rice in salted water.

Bake the asparagus in the oven, after having seasoned it with salt and olive oil. Cook the diced onion, together with the rosemary and the pine nuts into a heated pan, with olive oil. Take the salmon and cook it in another heated pan. Serve the salmon with brown rice, asparagus and pine nuts. Enjoy!

- Peach, mango and banana smoothie
  - Ingredients required – protein powder (1 ½ scoops), peach (1/2 cup), mango (1/2 cup), banana (1/2), organic milk (1 cup), ice cubes (4)
  - Preparation - add all the above mentioned ingredients into your blender and process them until they are thoroughly mixed. Pour the contents into a large glass and enjoy.

- Cranberry, spinach and quinoa salad
  - Ingredients required – quinoa (2 cups, cooked), spinach (2 cups), cranberries (1/4

cup), pears (2), walnuts (1/4 cup), apple cider vinegar (1 ½ tbsp.), extra virgin olive oil (2 tbsp.), salt and pepper to taste

- o Preparation – take a large bowl and add the following ingredients together: quinoa, spinach, cranberries, pear slices and walnuts. Prepare the dressing for the salad by mixing the apple cider vinegar with the extra virgin olive oil (adding salt and pepper to taste). Toss the salad in order to distribute the dressing in an even manner and refrigerate before serving. Enjoy!

- Chocolate almond butter
  - o Ingredients required – banana (1, frozen), almond milk (1 cup), almond butter (1/2 tbsp.), protein powder (1 scoop, chocolate flavor)
  - o Preparation - add all the above mentioned ingredients into your blender and process them until they are thoroughly mixed. Pour the contents into a large glass and enjoy.

These are just several recipes you can consider in order to prevent or revert the negative effects of leptin-resistance. As you have seen for yourself, all of these recipes include healthy food choices, activating the metabolism and promoting the weight loss.

Chapter 7 – Top things to remember about leptin resistance

Leptin is the satiety hormone, playing an essential role in the control of the appetite. It is also the hormone that allows for the weight to remain within normal limits, as it sends to the brain the full signal. More recent studies have shown that the leptin hormone is also capable of stimulating the sympathetic nervous system, which actually lead to the burning of the excess adipose tissue.

In the situation that a person has developed leptin resistance, this means that the body has increased quantities of leptin circulating in the blood and in different organs but the body simply does not respond to the activity of the leptin. In case you are wondering why leptin resistance occurs, you should know that there is more than one hypothesis proposed by the specialists in the healthcare field.

Some studies have demonstrated that the leptin hormone does not reach the brain, so as to provide it with the full signal (no control of the appetite, which leads to overeating and weight gain). Other studies have blamed the leptin resistance on the receptors that leptin should bind to. They consider that, when these receptors do not function properly, the activity of the leptin hormone is inhibited. The latter theory has been often associated with those who are overweight or obese; it is considered that once the activity of the leptin hormone is inhibited, the control of the appetite is impossible and thus the weight gain occurs.

When the body has developed resistance to leptin, the person will start to experience frequent cravings or feel hungry all the time. As you have seen, the leptin diet is essential, in order to control these cravings and be successful in the weight loss process. The leptin resistance often appears as the result of long-term bad eating habits, such as the consumption of high fructose corn syrup or increased quantities of carbohydrates. It should also be noted that the leptin resistance is not only caused by the inadequate diet but also by other habits that are not that good either, including the constant stress or the lack of sleep.

Fortunately, the leptin resistance can be prevented or reverted by changing the way you eat. In the anterior chapters, you have had the opportunity to read about the leptin diet and the way it can help you lose weight. One of the most important things to remember about this diet is that it is mainly based on protein and fiber intake, this helping you to keep your cravings under control.

If you want to prevent or revert the leptin resistance, you must always think whether the food you are eating is a healthy choice or not. As you move on from the protein/fiber mix powder meals and resume your three meals per day, you have to pay attention to the things you are eating. The healthy choices are often the most obvious ones – for example, you can always choose oatmeal for breakfast, as this will provide your body with everything it needs (helping the leptin hormone send the satiety signal to the brain). The same goes for peanut butter – this is an excellent source of healthy proteins and it has also been shown to reduce the cravings or hunger sensation.

As it can be quite difficult to give up bad habits and start afresh, with a new diet, you can ease your stress by taking natural supplements. These are going to help you with the weight loss process, ensuring a status of optimal health at the same time. One of the most recommended supplements for those who are experiencing leptin resistance is the one that contains African mango extract. Studies performed on overweight and obese participants have shown that the supplements that contain this natural extract are capable of improving the leptin sensitivity; moreover, they allow for the body weight to be kept under control (together with the diet and the physical exercise).

At the level of the brain, keep in mind that the leptin hormone acts on the receptors that are found in the hypothalamus. The activity of the leptin hormone is essential for the regulation of the appetite and the homeostasis of the body, as you have probably understood by now. The leptin hormone has a dual functioning mechanism – on one hand, it acts on the receptors that are found at the level of the lateral hypothalamus, inhibiting the hunger sensation; on the other hand, it influences the receptors of the medial hypothalamus, stimulating the satiety sensation (hence its name).

Always remember that, in healthy individuals, the levels of circulating levels in the blood are at their highest point during the night. These levels are so high, so that they suppress the appetite, allowing the body to rest and benefit from the rejuvenating sleep. The blood leptin levels follow a diurnal rhythm and this can be easily disturbed by the leptin resistance. Fortunately, leptin resistance is not a problem that cannot be solved. The leptin diet, based on the careful timing of the meals, remains the best choice for those who want to revert the effects of the leptin resistance.

In more recent studies, it has been found that the high levels of triglycerides (commonly found in those who are either overweight or obese) are responsible for the leptin not reaching its target. When there are too many triglycerides circulating in the blood (due to the constant eating or snacking), the transfer of leptin across the blood circulation is simply impaired and the brain does not receive the full or satiety signal (hence the overeating and the weight gain). In many people, the problem is made even worse, as the leptin resistance is aggravated by the post-leptin receptor deficit.

These are the most important things that you need to remember about the leptin resistance and how it can influence your weight. Use this information in order to understand what happens inside your body and do not hesitate to try out the leptin diet, so as to revert the effects of the leptin resistance.

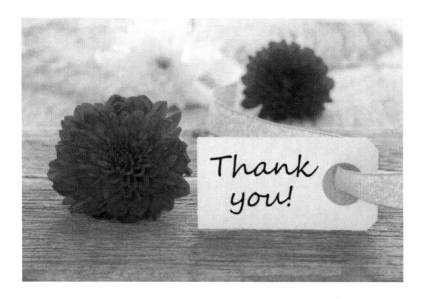

Finally, if you enjoyed this book, then I'd like to ask you for a favor, would you be kind enough to leave a review for this book on Amazon? It'd be greatly appreciated!

Thank you and good luck!

Printed in Great Britain
by Amazon